Pascal Zéphirin KABANGU TSHILA

OXYTOCYN INFUSION DELIVERY IN KISANGANI

Pascal Zéphirin KABANGU TSHILA

OXYTOCYN INFUSION DELIVERY IN KISANGANI

ScienciaScripts

Imprint

Cover image: www.ingimage.com

This book is a translation from the original published under ISBN 978-613-9-53189-9.

Publisher:
Sciencia Scripts
is a trademark of
Dodo Books Indian Ocean Ltd. and OmniScriptum S.R.L publishing group

120 High Road, East Finchley, London, N2 9ED, United Kingdom
Str. Armeneasca 28/1, office 1, Chisinau MD-2012, Republic of Moldova, Europe
Managing Directors: Ieva Konstantinova, Victoria Ursu
info@omniscriptum.com

Printed at: see last page
ISBN: 978-620-8-54653-3

DEDICATION

- To my mother Marie Jeanne MIKITSHI ETOBO for all the sacrifice, affection and love shown to us from the moment we were conceived until now. May poverty be neither an end nor a disaster, for the family of which you are the architect will make your face shine for those who have never known you;

- To all my brothers and sisters;

- To all the family Jean Pierre ETOBO

- To my wife Sara Yvonne KABIKA

- To my children : Maxime TsHILA KABANGU, Nolan ETOBO KABANGU, Rayan MAKETCHI KABANGU

- To all my loved ones;

I dedicate this work, the fruit of so many sacrifices.

Zéphyrin Pascal KABANGU TSHILA

ACKNOWLEDGEMENTS

- *Our deepest gratitude goes first of all to the Eternal God of all grace, the sole designer and maker of all that we are.*

- *We would also like to express our gratitude to Professor Emmanuel KOMANDA LIKWEKWE and Doctor Jeannine NADI, respectively director and supervisor of this work, for having accepted to direct and supervise this work despite their multiple occupations. Their opinions, considerations and remarks edified us throughout this work, and we will never forget their remarks, which were addressed rigorously but with a kind attitude towards us.*

- *We would also like to thank our uncle, Jean Pierre Etobo, for the love and availability he has shown us by supporting our studies from beginning to end, and we would like to express our deep gratitude to him;*

- *Our thanks go to all the heroes behind the scenes who supported us both morally and materially in carrying out this work: Kally KALONJI, Sheila SHILO, Justine TSHIDIBI, Gaston TSHIBAKA, Jean Pierre KIBAMBI, Willy NGOYI, Gilbert MALANGO*

- *We would also like to thank our uncle Albert NSHISU and our big brother Léonard TSHIKUDI for their sense of being and their great generosity.*

- *We would also like to thank all who, from near and far, have supported us morally and materially throughout our academic career. Our thoughts are with the families of Alden KALEMBO, Adolphe NTAMBWE, Nico NYONGONI, Jean MULONGO and others.*

- *All the fellow students in this year's class, with whom we have shared some of the most difficult and, no doubt, some of the most enjoyable moments of our university life.*

- *Finally, to all those who contributed in one way or another to the development of this work and who have not been mentioned, we say a big thank you.*

Zephyrin Pascal KABANGU TSHILA

0.INTRODUCTION

0.1. ISSUES

In normal childbirth, the live foetus is expelled through the natural birth canal by the force of uterine contractions alone, aided in the final moments by abdominal effort. Natural childbirth therefore requires no intervention, whether medicinal, manual or instrumental. The doctor's role was limited to waiting and monitoring, whereas nowadays he or she intervenes before, during and after childbirth with increasing frequency [16].

Let's say that childbirth comes naturally after about 41 weeks of amenorrhoea. That's around 9 and a half months or 283 days (from the date of your last period). The normal term of delivery is from the beginning of the 37th week to the end of the 41st week. Below this, the term is premature, and above thisoverdue. It is fair to ask whether labour accelerated by an oxytocin infusion can be considered eutoctopic [1]. It should be remembered that a delivery is said to be eutoctal when it occurs at term in a pregnancy which has progressed normally with the onset of labour in a pregnancy which has progressed normally with the onset of spontaneous labour, and when it progresses normally without instrumental intervention [23]. MANGA adds to these criteria: the child must be in cephalic vertex presentation and the delivery must be vaginal and live [14]. When a delivery meets all these criteria, it is termed an eutoctopic delivery. If it does not, it is dystocic [23]. Dystocia is characterised by the opposite: irregularity, excess, difficulty or cessation of physiological phenomena [16].

In the light of the above, we can understand that childbirth by oxytocin infusion is not a "cure-all". eutocique childbirth, on the other hand, medical childbirth (oxytocin infusion...) is a method based on medicinal actions to correct anomalies, and therefore certain standards of dynamic dystocies [16]: "inefficient uterine activity, hypokinesia, localised disorders of uterine activity:

localised insufficiencies of uterine contraction, localised body contractions or DEMELIN syndrome,...". [12]. Oxytocics, taken in their etymological sense, make childbirth faster. However, this term refers to drugs which strengthen uterine contraction. Syntocinon is therefore used during labour exclusively by the IV route in 5% isotonic glucose serum solutions. Several preparations can be used: 5 to 10 units in 500 ml if syntocinon is used with a volumetric pump (which should be preferred to the dropper during live birth). Although the importance of the start and doses of syntocinon in the treatment of dynamic dystocia has been the subject of controversy, several protocols for its use have been proposed [21].

There are several reasons why obstetricians now induce labour in certain pregnant women, and a number of techniques have been developed to induce labour, including the infusion of oxytocin [27].

Worldwide, there are two situations in childbirth is induced: either at the request of the mother-to-be and/or the doctor, or in a medical emergency [22].

The retrospective study by WEIN in 1989 confirms the data according to which 1220 artificial labour inductions for myotomy and continuous oxytocin infusion were performed [21]. In France, the study conducted by Julia BLANCHOT at Paris Descartes University in 2011 on artificial induction of labour at term at Port-Royal showed that 39.9% of Induction of labour has been achieved with oxytocin infusion and various indications have been selected [10].

Data on the use of oxytocics in Africa are very limited. However, wide variations in the frequency of oxytocin use during the periods of effacement, dilation and expulsion were observed in 1998 in several African countries: in Senegal with a frequency of 2.5% in Kaolack and 32.9% in St Louis, in Burkina Faso (Ouagadougou) with 10.5% in Mauritania (Nouakchott) with 13.0% in Niger (Niamey) with 5.7% in Mali (Bamako) with 26,1% in Côte d'Ivoire (Abidjan) with 13.4% and in 2000 in Napal (Katmandu) with 31.1% (18.30), in

2010 at the Hôpital de la Mère et de l'Enfant Lagune (HOMEL) in Cotonou (BENIN) with 8.4% [19].

Developing countries, like other regions of the world, face the challenge of making the best use of limited resources to improve the health of women and children. Obstetric interventions should be evidence-based, and interventions that are effective only for high-risk groups should not be used routinely [30]. However, excessive oxytocin administration can cause hyperstimulation, uterine hypertonia [18], uterine hyperkinesiasperineal tearing, fetal heart rate abnormalities and meconium amniotic fluid failure [10].

In DR Congo, a study carried out in Kinshasa in 2004 by KANGUDIA et . "Sur l'induction du travail d'accouchement en milieux sous équipés" showed that induction of labour by oxytocin infusion is practised both in primiparous and multiparous women, and the reasons for these indications for labour were varied. In Kisangani, data on delivery by oxytocin infusion are very few or even almost non-existent, and if they do exist, they are very old. In a study of pregnant women with prolonged pregnancies in the CUKIS, he found that 62.5% of pregnant women benefited from an oxytocin infusion associated or not with amniotomy to induce labour (11;5). It is therefore due to the lack of clear and reliable data on the frequency and main indications for the use of oxytocin infusion in childbirth in our environment that we have taken on the task of writing this report. The main advantage of oxytocin infusion is not only its route of administration [11]. It also legitimate to use it because it is the cheapest and best controlled method, with the fewest side-effects [9].

The objectives of induction vary according to the indication: in medical indications, the aim is reduce foetomaternal morbidity and mortality [25].

The problem with oxytocin infusion delivery is that obviously all accidents are possible and are sometimes attributed to the induction, i.e. the obstetrician, and not to the delivery itself. However, these accidents seem to occur more frequently [14]. At the end of this reflection, we ask ourselves the following questions: what are the main indications for induction of labour by oxytocin infusion in our environment, i.e. in Kisangani, how often is labour artificially induced by this method and what are the complications arising from it? This research will attempt to answer these questions.

0.2. OBJECTIVE AND PURPOSE OF THE WORK

Throughout our study, we will seek to identify the problem of oxytocin infusion in Kisangani with a view to improving the management of pregnant women.

0.2.1. SPECIFIC OBJECTIVES

- Determining the frequency of delivery by oxytocin infusion in Kisangani;
- Identify the main indications;
- Determine the complications arising from it.

0.3. INTEREST OF THE WORK

The importance of this work is such that it enables us to identify the most frequent indications requiring oxytocin infusion in childbirth in our environment, and to remind practitioners of advantages and disadvantages of this practice.

0.4. WORK SUBDIVISIONS

The present work is divided into four chapters, of which, apart from the introduction :

- The first deals with general information on oxytocin infusion delivery;
- The second presents materials and methods;
- The third section presents the results, comments and discussion.

Finally, we will conclude with some suggestions.

CHAPTER I

GENERAL INFORMATION

I. DEFINITION OF CONCEPTS

1.1.DELIVERY

Childbirth is the set of mechanical and physiological phenomena which result in the exit of the foetus and its appendages from the maternal genital tract, from 22 weeks onwards. For delivery to occur, the foetal mobile must progress through the pelvic-genital tract under the influence of uterine contractions. [12].

1.2.THE OCYTOCINES

Oxytocins are substances which, like oxytocin, cause the uterine muscle to contract after it has been impregnated with oestrogen during pregnancy. [15]. Oxytocin, also known as oxytocin, a polypeptide made up of nine amino acids. It is synthesised in the supraoptic and paraventricular nuclei of the hypothalamus, transported and stored in secretory granules. This hormone stimulates uterine contractions in pregnant women and accelerates labour during childbirth. [27].

II. GENERAL CONSIDERATIONS

2.1.Assessment of uterine contractions

During labour, the CUs can be measured and qualified. We can then accurately describe their frequency, total intensity (maximum pressure recorded), true intensity (total intensity minus base tone), duration and base tone (lowest pressure between ECs). Their frequency increases from 1 every 15-20 minutes to 3-4 every 10 minutes before expulsion. Their intensity, duration and frequency also increase between the beginning and end of labour. Lindgren proved that cervical dilation only began if the intensity of the contractions was high enough to ensure good uterine dynamics.

During labour, EC is intermittent, total and involves entire uterine muscle. Between beginning and end of labour, EC varies considerably. Tocography is used to assess them.

Two methods can be used to measure contractions:

- The first is external tocography, the most widely used in France. It consists of a capsule containing a spring, placed at the level of the uterine fundus, which enables the intensity and basic tone to be determined.
- The second method is internal tocography. This is a semi-invasive method requiring prior rupture of the membranes and 2 cm dilatation. It is used as a second-line method, because of the risk of infection, to measure the true intensity of contractions and their basic tone, and thus make a better diagnosis of dynamic abnormalities.

The unit of measurement for CU is the Montevideo unit (UM), expressed in kPa/15min. The pressure curve qualifying the contraction is asymmetrical, with descending relaxation phase. Between two contractions, it is essential for the uterus to relax completely, in order to regain its resting tone.

The vaginal touch cannot be used to measure or qualify EC, but it can be used to assess its effectiveness. Evaluation of EC and vaginal touch allow us to diagnose abnormalities. [10,11].

2.2. ANOMALIES AT WORK REQUIRING THE USE OF OXYTOCIN

Any abnormality occurring during labour should be the subject of a precise aetiological investigation, such as mechanical dystocia, dynamic dystocia and abnormal cervical dilatation. We will begin by discussing dynamic dystocia in general, then go on to look in more detail at induction dystocia and dystocia during labour. Finally, we will discuss disorders of uterine dynamics. [17].

2.2.1. Dynamic dystocies

2.2.1.1. Definitions

Dynamic dystocia is any contractile anomaly. It refers to "all the phenomena that disrupt the functioning of the uterine muscle during labour contractions, which may result in inefficient cervical dilatation" (Magnin). It corresponds an abnormality in uterine contraction and results in dilatation. < 1cm/h, whereas the normal rate of dilation is 1cm/h or more. In the presence of abnormal cervical dilatation, the first thing to rule out is mechanical dystocia. This is indicated by a fetopelvic presentation (FPD), a shrunken pelvis and/or macrosomia and an abnormal or malflexed presentation. We then look for dynamic dystocia. [3, 10]

2.2.1.2. Circumstances of discovery

Dynamic dystocia is diagnosed by analysing the partogram. It shows a defect, slow or stagnant dilatation, an abnormal partogram, a defect in the progression of the presentation and an abnormal EC. UC abnormalities can also be detected by monitoring or palpation. Once an anomaly has been discovered, it is essential to analyse it in order to qualify it. This analysis is carried out using several methods. [17].

2.2.1.3. Analysis methods

The CU correspond to the subjective painful sensations felt by the parturient, the periodicity and the increasingly short duration. The objective clinic uses the operator's hand to palpate these same parameters. The external tocographic recording assesses the The frequency of contractions and internal tocography provide information about the real intensity of the contractions, their duration and their basic tone. Analysis methods will enable dynamic dystocies to be classified into two groups: induction dystocies and dystocies during labour, which we will discuss. [20].

2.2.2. Starting dystocies

This name was given by Lacomme to situations where there is an absence of cervical dilation in women, often primiparous women, with painful and poorly tolerated contractions which do not give way spontaneously. Start-up dystocia is often linked to the anxiety and agitation caused by EC. Contractions are irregular, put pressure on the cervix poorly and are 5 minutes or more apart. The length of the latency phase varies according to the conditions of admission. If the latency phase is longer than 20 hours for a nulliparous mother and 14 hours for a mutiparous mother, Friedman refers to this as induction dystocia. According to the WHO (World Health Organisation), the latency phase must be greater than 8 hours in order to speak of incipient dystocia. The more mature the cervix at the start of labour, the shorter the duration of the latency phase. The height of the presentation at the start of labour seems to be a predictive factor for dystocia. If the presentation is high in a nulliparous woman, the caesarean section rate seems to be increased, unlike in a multiparous woman. Start-up dystocia is most often diagnosed on the basis of the partogram, which shows the absence or slowness of cervical dilatation. They are also diagnosed by tocography, which shows hypokinesia of frequency or irregularity of EC. Treatment of these dystocies differs depending on whether the cervix is rigid with dilatation< to 2cm, or whether the cervix is virtually effaced, flexible with dilatation to 2cm. When the cervix is rigid and dilated by more than 2cm, soothing treatment is recommended. This does not require an infusion of Syntocinon. If the cervix is virtually effaced, supple and dilated to 2cm, an infusion of Syntocinon is required, following epidural analgesia, to regulate the EC and make it more effective on the cervix. When contractions occur every 2 to 3 minutes, the membranes can be artificially ruptured if this has not happened spontaneously. Start-up dystocies are not the only dynamic dystocies; there are also dystocies during labour.

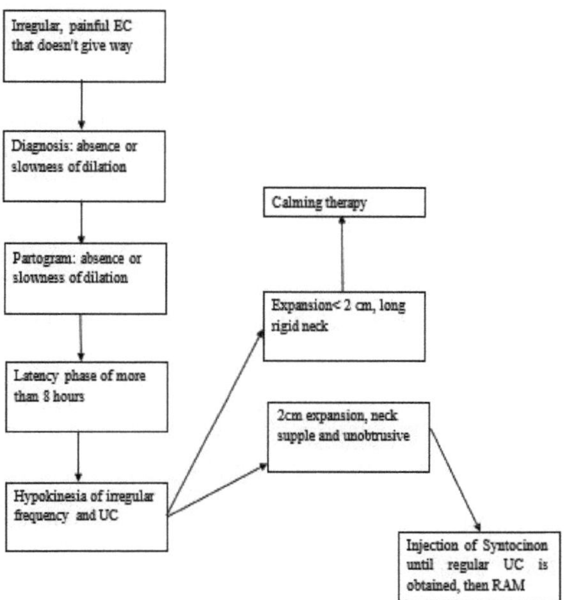

2.2.3. Dystocies during labour

This is a stagnation of dilatation at a time when the patient is clearly in labour, when she has entered the active phase. This is diagnosed by the partogram, which shows a horizontal dilatation curve. During the first stage of labour, hypokinesias can be observed. Dystocia can also be diagnosed in the second stage of labour.

2.2.3.1. Hypokinesia

Hypokinesia is responsible for 30% of dilatation anomalies. This anomaly results in regular but insufficiently frequent CU, with two contractions more than 3 minutes apart, lasting< to 70 seconds and of intensity< 30 mmHg. This results in cervical dilatation< 1 cm/h. It may be of primary origin (large multiparity, uterine malformation, uterine fibroid) or secondary (dystocic presentation, DFP, prævia obstacle, uterine overdistension, poorly flexed presentation, epidural analgesia (EPA) too early, excessive use of sedatives or analgesia).Hypokinesia leads to long, tiring labour and often instrumental extractions, as well as maternal-foetal infections, stained amniotic fluid (AF)abnormalities in the foetal heart rate (FHR) linked to foetal distress and foetal hypoxia.

Active management of labour is then indicated in the absence of obstetric criteria with a poor prognosis, such as macrosomia, pathological pelvis, signs of mechanical dystocia (large serosanguineous bump, onset of suture overlap) and very high presentation.

Labour is induced by artificial rupture of the membranes (AMR), followed by an oxytocin infusion if there is no response 30 to 60 minutes after AMR. Oxytocin is used to induce uterine contractions every 2 to 3 minutes. If the foetal presentation is very high, A Syntocinon infusion is recommended before performing AMR, due to the risk of cord procidence. Amniotomy can be performed with caution one hour later, even if the presentation remains identical. When the EC seems sufficient but dilation is not progressing, it is recommended that an internal tocography be installed to check the intensity of the contractions.

Labour management (amniotomy and use of oxytocics) can reduce labour time in the event of abnormal dilatation, ensuring correct uterine dynamics and resumption of dilatation. This has been confirmed by numerous studies. In any case, if dilation still does not exceed 1 cm/hour despite correct dynamics, the problem of EPD or malflexed presentation should be raised again, and an obstetrician should be called in. If dilation remains unchanged for 2 hours, even if the FFR is correct, caesarean section is recommended.

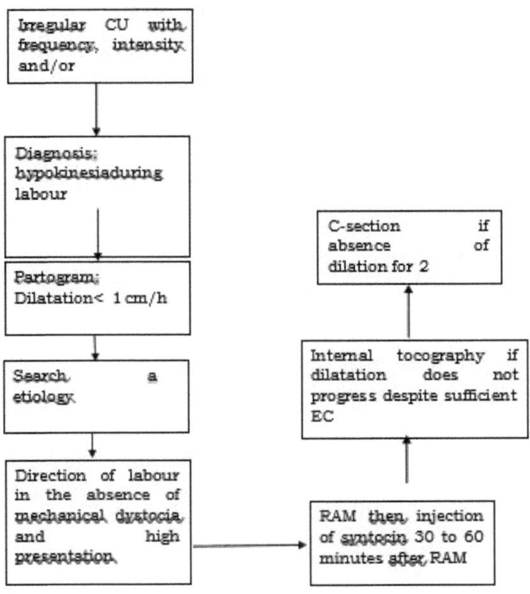

2.3.3.2 Dystocia in the second phase of labour

The progress of labour during this phase is measured in terms of descent and rotation of the presentation. Rotation of the fetal head is necessary for the presentation to descend into the pelvis. Dystocia in the second stage of labour occurs when the engagement and descent of the presentation is too slow. The foetal presentation must engage, descend and disengage within two hours of full dilation. This type of dystocia also occurs when the presentation does not progress for 45 minutes after full dilation. The aetiologies are macrosomia, PFD and dystocic presentations (posterior presentation, breech presentation, transverse presentation, deflexed presentation). Oxytocin can transform a difficult rotation forceps into an easy extraction, or even a spontaneous birth, as the increased intensity of contractions promotes rotation. If presentation does not progress for 30 minutes, an oxytocin infusion is recommended. If presentation persists beyond 60 minutes of maximum-dose oxytocin infusion, a caesarean section is recommended. Directed labour would slightly reduce the caesarean section rate, but not all authors are unequivocal. During dynamic dystocia, it is important to monitor the progress of dilatation or fetal presentation as well as the tocography, as disturbances in the rhythm of EC may appear. [17, 12, 9, 16].

2.3.3.3 Uterine contractility disorders

Normally uterine contractility is regular from the onset of labour. However, there are rhythm abnormalities, and bi- or trigeminal contractions can sometimes be observed, i.e. two or three successive contractions which are not separated by a return to basic tone between each contraction. This situation is dangerous when oxytocin is used, as there is a risk of hypertonia. The tracing may become anarchic, with no precise rhythm. Contractions follow one another and dilation is slow or stopped.

Traditionally, oxytocics have been used to treat uterine contractility disorders. However, it would appear that this is not the right treatment, as some of these irregularities border on hypertonia. It would therefore be more advisable to use mimetics, which are utero-relaxing. Insufficient uterine contractions at the start of or during labour, or dynamic or mechanical dystocia, must be identified. and corrected. Whether dynamic or mechanical, it is the leading cause of caesarean sections in primiparous women. Early correction of uterine contractility deficiencies is the principal means reducing the duration of labour through continuous intravenous infusion of oxytocin. Syntocinon is a first-line treatment for reinforcing the frequency and intensity of uterine contractions during the onset or activation of labour in order to reduce its duration.

2.3. Presentation of oxytocics

The oxytocics consist of oxytocin (international non-proprietary name). Oxytocin has been synthesised since 1953, its commercial name being Syntocinon. It is a natural hormone: oxytocin, which is identical to that produced by our body's hypothalamus. Oxytocics are powerful uterotonics that increase the contractile force of the uterus and regulate EC. Syntocinon has been marketed since 13 August 1970 (date of marketing authorisation). Studies show that early and systematic direction is more detrimental to labour than non-systematic direction, since it does not offer any advantages in terms duration of labour, foetal and maternal condition, or the number of vaginal deliveries, even though a slight reduction in the caesarean section rate has been demonstrated in several studies. These studies are not all unequivocal. The prescription of Syntocinon should therefore not be systematic, but should follow a medical indication in the context of directed work. [6, 17, 16].

2.3.1. Indications for the use oxytocin

The direction of labour during childbirth is indicated in the presence of dynamic dystocia either at the beginning or during labour. Oxytocin is also indicated in the event of malflexion of the foetal presentation and dystocia of the second stage of labour. Directed labour thus makes it possible to reduce the diameter of foetal engagement. Labour that has been induced artificially on a mature cervix can also be directed. An epidural is not an indication for a Syntocinon infusion. The indications for labour, as well as the contraindications, which we discuss below, must be respected.

2.3.2. Contraindications to supervised work

These contraindications are linked to the injection of oxytocin. There are absolute and relative contraindications. Absolute contraindications include PPD, previa obstructions and dystocic presentation (front or transverse), previous foetal distress or distress in early labour, uterine hypertonicity when delivery is not imminent and hypersensitivity to the drug. Relative contraindications include scarred uteri, high multiparity, breech presentation, multiple pregnancies, hydramnios, cardiovascular disorders, severe arterial hypertension (AH), predisposition to amniotic embolisms (in-utero foetal death and retroplacental haematoma). However, it is often possible to carry out directed labour despite the presence of relative contraindications, with the help of reinforced and more attentive monitoring. If oxytocin is injected incorrectly or in the presence of contraindications, adverse effects may occur. [17].

2.3.3. Undesirable effects

Injecting oxytocin can have an impact on the uterus, on the general state of the parturient and on the foetus.

2.3.3.1. General effects

When the dose of oxytocin injected is very high, arterial hypotensionand a tachycardia followed by arterial hypertension (AH), bradycardia and increased central venous pressure. In the case of a massive dose of Syntocinon (greater than 120 mU/min, when 50 to 80 mU/min should not be exceeded), an antidiuretic effect will appear, manifested by transient water intoxication. This is rare but serious, and is linked to a massive intake of oxytocin and oxytocic dilution solution. This intoxication leads to nausea, vomiting and headaches, followed by a coma with convulsions and hyponatremia. Exceptionally, a rash, an anaphylactoid reaction or anaphylactic shock may occur.

2.3.3.2. Uterine effects

Syntocinon can cause uterine hyperstimulation. This takes the form of hyperkinesia and/or frequency. A high dose will lead to an increase in the resting tone of the UC. This is known as uterine hyperkinesia or hypertonia. Uterine rupture may also occur, although this is exceptional, but the risk is increased in the case of a scarred uterus. The administration of oxytocin should be monitored by internal tocography in the presence of a scarred uterus, especially as the same dose has variable effects from one person to another.

2.3.3.3. Foetal effects

Acute foetal distress may be the result of uterine hypertonia or hyperkinesia. Early, systematic amniotomy and/or the administration of high doses of oxytocin are associated with disturbances in FCR. Such practices therefore require a great deal of caution and monitoring. Syntocinon also appears to be indirectly responsible for neonatal hyperbilirubinemia. Oxytocin is thought to weaken foetal red blood cells under the effect of Syntocinon-induced hypo-osmolarity. However, this anomaly is found in the presence of long labour, a serosanguineous bump or a cephalohaematoma. Syntocinon is therefore not the only cause of hyperbilirubinaemia. This pathophysiology is not unequivocal for everyone. [17, 27].

2.4. Administration of Syntocinon

The administration of Syntocinon includes its presentation, route of administration, dosage, drug interactions and prescription.

2.4.1. Preparing the Syntocinon infusion

Syntocinon is a commercial solution in the form of a 1 ml ampoule containing 5 international units (IU) of oxytocin and excipients (sodium acetate, chlorobutanol, ethyl alcohol, acetic acid and water for injection). It should be stored in a refrigerator at a temperature of between +2°C and +8°C. The ampoule is diluted in isotonic saline or 5% glucose. A 5IU ampoule is usually diluted in 500 ml. It can also be diluted in 49 ml of 5% isotonic glucose if administered using a 50 ml electric syringe. The administration of oxytocin requires uterine and foetal monitoring from the moment the infusion is started until delivery, in order to detect foetal distress or a uterine anomaly at an early stage. The infusion of Syntocinon should be placed as a bypass to a maintenance infusion (containing saline), as no other substance should be added to Syntocinon. When combined with other drugs, the rate of oxytocin infusion may be increased. However, oxytocin should be administered at a controlled rate and increased cautiously until good uterine dynamics are achieved.

2.4.2. Drug interactions

During or after PDA, oxytocin may potentiate the vasoconstrictive effect of sympathomimetics. Certain volatile anaesthetics such as cyclopropane or halothane may aggravate the hypotensive effect of oxytocin and reduce its uterotonic action. In the event of concomitant administration, foetal and maternal rhythm disorders may occur. Prostaglandins may also potentiate the effect of oxytocin. In order to avoid the appearance of drug interactions or undesirable effects, and thus to ensure the safety of the work, not all healthcare professionals are authorised to prescribe Syntocinon. [27].

2.5. PARTICULAR SITUATION

Macrosomia, PFD, scar uterus, fever in early labour, tinted LA, hypertension, breech presentation and delivery of twins are all situations that may require oxytocin infusion during labour, despite relative contraindication, as they favour anomalies.

2.5.1. Delivery of a macrosomic fetus or trial of labour for fetopelvic disproportion

This situation leads to dilatation anomalies. Only hyporcinesia justifies treatment with an oxytocin infusion. This infusion must be started very carefully, as studies have shown that the rate of shoulder dystocia doubles in foetuses weighing over 4500g, where dilation has stopped or is abnormally slow during labour. Care must therefore be taken not to force cephalic presentation.

2.5.2. Scarred uterus

In this situation, hypokinesia is the most frequent cause of abnormal dilatation. Uterine dynamics are monitored by external tocography for as long as the membranes remain. When a dilatation anomaly is diagnosed, internal tocography is recommended to qualify and treat hypokinesia (of frequency and/or intensity).The indicated treatment is an infusion of Syntocinon, following AMR, only if there is maximum surveillance and without ever exceeding a flow rate of 20 Mui/h. Any intervention (AMR and/or infusion of Syntocinon) must result in resumption of dilation within the hour, as stagnation of dilation is not accepted beyond 2 hours. If there is a sudden change in uterine activity (hyper or hyperkinesia), uterine rupture must be considered immediately, as hyperkinesia in a scarred uterus is the first sign of scar dehiscence. In the event of hyperkinesia, the best course of action is to inform the doctor and prepare the woman for an emergency caesarean section.

2.5.3. Fever at the start of labour

Dysregulation of the thermoregulatory centre follows an ovarian, extra-ovarian or generalised maternal infection. 20% of febrile women give birth to infected foetuses. There are risks for the foetus (neonatal infections, foetal suffering, prematurity, increased perinatal mortality, respiratory distress and intra-ventricular haemorrhage), for the mother (endometritis, bacteraemia, septicaemia, toxic and infectious shock, and coagulopathy), and labour (increased duration of labour, foetal suffering, increased rate of caesarean section and instrumental extraction).One of the treatments for fever in early labour is dilation. This corrects dynamic dystocia and reduces the duration of labour, thereby reducing the risks for the mother and foetus and reducing labour abnormalities.

2.5.4. Tinted amniotic fluid

This leads to foetal inhalation and infection, as well as abnormal fetal heart rhythms. Directing labour therefore helps to limit these pathologies. When the LA is tinted but transparent, the progress of labour should be monitored, especially the FHR, and labour should be directed if an abnormality in the progress of labour is diagnosed. When the LA is meconium, the ECR is often normal or only slightly pathological. In favourable local conditions, labour should be directed. In the presence of pathological LA, labour must be rapid in order to reduce the risk of meconium inhalation and foetal infection. This treatment requires maximum surveillance using monitoring, saturometry and pH at the scalp.

2.5.5. Known and suspected hypertension

The presence of hypertension in early labour must be managed with caution. Labour and delivery require a minimum of force. The duration of expulsive efforts should therefore be limited. The risk of hypertonia, tachysystole or hypersystole in the foetus means that the dynamics of labour must be monitored more closely.

2.5.6. Presentation of the headquarters

The diagnosis of breech presentation is generally made during pregnancy, more rarely during labour. risks incurred during delivery asphyxia, trauma, procidence of the cord, difficulties in extraction due to retention of the last head or extension of the arms. The VBAC must take place in safe conditions: the obstetrician must be on site and it must be possible to perform a caesarean section as quickly as possible. The dilatation phase must regular and the RCF monitored at all times. The membranes must be kept intact for as long as possible. If hypokinesia is present, and only if there is no distress, an oxytocin infusion may be prescribed. Stagnation of dilation should not exceed 2 to 3 hours and the total duration of labour should not exceed 10 hours. The FHR should remain correct throughout labour. At the moment of expulsion, an oxytocin infusion is recommended to ensure that delivery is as rapid as possible.

2.5.7. vaginal delivery in twin pregnancies

These deliveries entail risks such as cord procidence, foetal asphyxiafoetal entanglement and cord entanglement. A vaginal delivery is possible if the first foetus is in cephalic presentation. Monitoring of the FHR of each twin is mandatory throughout labour, as is EC. Oxytocics may be used to regulate EC. Cervical dilatation must be as rapid in both the latent and active phases as in a single pregnancy. Expulsion of the first twin is identical to that of a single foetus. Delivery of the second twin requires directed labour. Immediately after the birth of the first twin, the Syntocinon infusion should be stopped to check the presentation of the second twin.

There are several possibilities:

- The second twin is in cephalic presentation, and CU is expected to resume. If they are slow in coming, the Syntocinon infusion is resumed, and then a RAM of the second bag is performed carefully to avoid laterocidence or procidence of the cord. Expulsion is then carried out rapidly.
- The second twin is in breech presentation, and the Syntocinon infusion must be systematically repeated to obtain good uterine dynamics. RAM is then carefully performed.

Other presentations of the second twin require specialised manoeuvres and not an infusion of Syntocinon. [10, 22, 17].

CHAPTER II

METHODOLOGY

II.1. TYPE

We conducted a descriptive and retrospective study in the General Referral Hospitals of the City of Kisangani and at CUKIS, in the period 1 January 2011 to 31 December 2012.

II.2. DESCRIPTION OF THE ENVIRONMENT

We conducted our research in the town of Kisangani, capital of Province Orientale (now Tshopo province) the Democratic Republic of Congo.

The city is made up of six municipalities, including :

- The municipality of Kabondo
- The municipality of Kisangani
- The municipality of Lubunga
- The municipality of Makiso
- The commune of Mangobo
- The municipality of Tshopo

To carry out our study, we visited all the HGRs and the CUKISs and collected data from :

- HGR KABONDO
- HGR LUBUNGA
- HGR MAKISO
- HGR MANGOBO
- HGR TSHOPO
- THE CUKIS

Each of these hospitals has four basic departments: Surgery, Gynaecology and Obstetrics, Internal Medicine and Paediatrics. The obstetrics and gynaecology department was the target for data collection in this study.

II.3. POPULATION OF STUDY

The study population consisted of 4,785 participants who were admitted to the labour ward in the six HGRs and the CUKISs.

II.4. SAMPLE

Our sample consisted of all parturients in whom an oxytocin infusion was placed to facilitate delivery in the six maternity units, i.e. 157 parturients (3.28%).

II.5. INCLUSION CRITERIA

- Any parturient monitored in the labour ward of the Kisangani university hospitals and clinics concerned is given an oxytocin infusion;
- To have a file containing the information we need for our study;
- Have received an oxytocin infusion during childbirth.

II.6. PARAMETERS TO BE ANALYSED

For each parturient, the parameters were analysed:

- Identity of parturients ;
- Socio-demographic characteristics ;
- Obstetrical formula; maternal and foetal complications.

II.7. TECHNIQUE FOR COLLECTING DATA

In order to achieve our objectives, we chose the technique of documentary analysis based on the use of hospitalization registers and the records of parturients admitted for childbirth during the period of our study by completing the survey protocol.

II.8. SURVEY PROCEDURE/PLAN FOR COLLECTING DATA

To facilitate the collection of our data, we first went to the Gynaecological-Obstetrics Department to count all the cases admitted for childbirth during our study period, and then listed all the cases of childbirth in the register (and especially all cases of childbirth by oxytocin infusion). Finally, we went to the archive department to look for the files of the women listedespecially those who had given birth using oxytocin infusion.

II.9. ANALYSIS OF DATA

For the statistical analysis of our results, taking into account their nature, we used the percentage calculation for the counting according to the following formula : %= ni Nx 100

Or: %: percentage N: total workforce ni: partial workforce
To find the average age of our gestating females, we used the following formula:
A= X+Y2

or: A: Average age

X: Age of the lowest extreme Y: Age of highest extreme

II.10. PROCESSING OF DATA

Our data was entered and processed using Excel 2010 software.

II.11. DEFINITION OF CERTAIN VARIABLES USED

- Primipara: woman who has given birth once
- Multipare: woman who has given birth 2 to 5 times
- Large multiparous: a woman who has given birth to 6 or babies.

II.12. DIFFICULTY ENCOUNTERED

Collecting the data was not easy:

- The absence of certain data in patient files;

- The irregularity of archive services ;
- Discrepancies between registers and records, i.e. there are a number of cases in the patient register but no records;
- Patient records that are not updated...

CHAPTER III

PRESENTATION AND ANALYSIS OF RESULTS

III.1. frequency

The table: 1. FREQUENCY ACCOUCTION BY OCYTOCIN PERFYSION

Parturiente	TOTAL WORKFORCE	%
Delivered by oxytocin infusion. Delivered without oxytocin infusion	157 4628	3,28 96,71
Total	4785	100

During our study period, a total of 157 cases of pregnant women having benefited from an oxytocin infusion during childbirth were counted out of a total of 4785 cases of parturients who went to the various maternity units in the city to give birth, i.e. a frequency of 3.28%, as shown in the table above.

III.2. SOCIO-DEMOGRAPHIC CHARACTERISTICS

a) The age of women giving birth

Table 2 : AGE DISTRIBUTION OF PARTNERS WHO RECEIVED OCYTICIN PERFUSION DURING DELIVERY IN KISANGANI

AGE	TOTAL WORKFORCE	CASE OF PERFUSION	%
< 20 years old	417	30	19,13
20-24 years old	1830	45	28,66
25-29 years old	1725	40	25,47
30-34 years old	608	21	13,37
≥ 35 years old	205	21	13,37
Total	4785	157	100

This table shows that most parturients who gave birth with oxytocin infusion were between 20 and 24 years old (28.66%) and 25 and 29 years old. (25,47%).

b) The residential community for women giving birth

Table 3: BREAKDOWN BY PLACE OF ORIGIN OF PREGNANT CHILDREN WHO HAVE RECEIVED PERFUSION OF OXYTOCIN DURING CHILDBIRTH IN KISANGANI

PLACE OF PROVENANCE	N	F	%
C. MAKISO	852	24	15,28
C. MANGOBO	1008	35	22,29
C. KABONDO	1200	54	34,39
C. TSHOPO	497	17	10,82
C. LUBUNGA	200	4	2,54
C. KISANGANI	932	16	10,86
OUTSIDE KISANGANI	96	6	3,82
Total	4785	157	100

The table shows the following Most of our respondents come from the commune of KABONDO with 34.39% or 35 cases, followed by the commune of MANGOBO with 22.29% or 35 cases. The commune of LUBUNGA was the least represented with 2.54% or 4 cases.

c) Civil status of new mothers

Table 4: DISTRIBUTION ACCORDING TO CIVIL STATUS OF DELIVERIES WHO RECEIVED OCYTOCIN PERFUSION DURING DELIVERY IN KISANGANI

CIVIL STATUS	N	F	%
MARIEE	4572	149	94,90
CELIBATORY	231	8	5,10
Total	4785	157	100

This table shows that 94.90% or 149 pregnant women were married.

d) The profession of birth attendants

Table 5: BREAKDOWN BY PROFESSION OF BIRTHGIVERS WHO RECEIVED OCYTOCIN PERFUSION DURING DELIVERY IN KISANGANI

PROFESSION	N	F	%
STUDENT/HOUSEK	122	34	21,65
EEPER CIVIL	4183	83	52,86
SERVANT	107	10	6,40
SHOPKEEPER	315	20	12,73
ARTIST	15	1	0,63
SEAMSTRESS	43	9	5,73
Total	4785	157	100

The table shows that most of our mothers are housewives (83 cases, or 52.86%), followed by students (34 cases, or 21.65%).

e) Parity in childbirth

Table 6: BREAKDOWN BY PARITY OF DELIVERIES WHO RECEIVED OCYTOCIN PERFUSION DURING DELIVERY IN KISANGANI

PARITY	N	F	%
PRIMIPAROUS	2404	69	43,94
MULTIPAROUS	2280	77	43,06
LARGE MULTIPAROUS	101	11	7,00
Total	4785	157	100

The table shows that primiparous and multiparous cows have almost the same frequency, with 43.94% for primiparous cows and 43.06% for multiparous cows.

III.3. Indications for oxytocin infusion

Table 7: BREAKDOWN OF OCYTOCIN PERFUSION DURING DELIVERY BY INDICATION

INDICATION	F	%
HYPOCINESIA MIU RPM PROLOGE PREGNANCY GEMELLAR PREGNANCY SFC OTHER	67 46 19 9 7 5 4	42,64 29,29 12,10 5,73 4,52 3,18 2,54
Total	157	100

In terms of indications, the table shows that hypokinesia has a higher frequency than other indications, with 42.64%, followed by MIU with 29.29%. Other indications came in at 2.54%.

III.4. Complications recorded

Table 8: DISTRIBUTION ACCORDING TO COMPLICATIONS RECORDED DURING DELIVERY IN PARTNERS WHO BENEFITED FROM OCYTOCIN PERFUSION IN KISANGANI

Complications	F	%
Failure Perineal tear Hypertonia ARCF hyperkinesia No complications	6 9 5 2 3 132	3,82 5,73 3,18 1,27 1,93 84,07
Total	157	100

ARCF: foetal heart rhythm abnormalities The table shows the following:
Most of our respondents had no complications either during or after the oxytocin infusion (84.07%), 5.73% had perineal tears and 3.82% had failed.

III.5. Clinical condition at the time the infusion is started

III.5.a. The condition of the water sac

Table 9: DISTRIBUTION ACCORDING TO WATER POCKET STATUS OF PARTNERS WHO RECEIVED OCYTOCIN PERFUSION DURING DELIVERY IN KISANGANI

WATER POCKET	F	%
NOT ROMPED ROMPUE	92 65	58,59 41,41
Total	157	100

The table shows that 92 parturients (58.59%) still had their water bags intact when they arrived at the hospital and 65 pregnant women (41.41%) arrived with their water bags already ruptured.

III.5.b. The quality of uterine contractions

Table 10: BREAKDOWN BY UTERINE CONTRACTION CHARACTERISTICS OF PARTNERS WHO RECEIVED AN OCYTOCIN PERFUSION DURING DELIVERY IN KISANGANI

CONTRACTIONS UTERINES	F	%
ABSENT WEAK FORTES	41 71 44	26,11 45,22 28,67
Total	157	100

The table shows that 45.22% of our respondents (71 cases) had weak uterine contractions on admission, 28.67% (44 cases) had strong contractions and 26.11% (41 cases) had no uterine contractions.

III.5.c. The degree of cervical dilation

Table 11: BREAKDOWN BY STATE OF DILATATION OF THE COLUMN AT ADMISSION OF PARTNERS WHO RECEIVED OCYTOCIN PERFUSION DURING DELIVERY IN KISANNGANI

DILATATION	F	%
0 1-2 3-4 ≥ 5	0 22 40 95	0 14,03 25,47 60,50
Total	157	100

From this table we make the following observations: 60.50% of our respondents, i.e. 65 cases, had cervical dilatation of more than 5 cm, followed by 25.47%, i.e. 40 cases, with dilatation between 3-4 cm and finally 14.03%, i.e. 22 cases with dilatation between 1-2 cm.

III.5.d. state of cervical effacement

Table 12: BREAKDOWN ACCORDING TO THE STATUS OF COLUMN EFFECTION OF PARTNERS WHO RECEIVED OCYTOCIN PERFUSION DURING DELIVERY IN KISANGANI

EFFACEMENT	F	%
0-30 40-50 60-70 ≥80	24 49 27 57	15,28 31,21 17,19 36,32
Total	157	100

This table shows that 36.32%, i.e. 57 parturients, had a cervical effacement of more than 80% on admission, followed by 31.21%, i.e. 49 cases with an effacement of between 40-50%, and 15.28%, i.e. 24 cases with an effacement of between 0-30%.

III.5.e. BCF status

Table XII: BREAKDOWN BY FETUS BCF OF PARTNERS WHO RECEIVED OCYTOCIN PRFUSION DURING DELIVERY IN KISANGANI

BCF	F	%
ABSENT	18	11,46
≤120 120-160	1	0,63
≥160	136	86,62
	2	1,29
Total	157	100

From this table we can see that 86.62% of the foetuses had BCFs present and between 120-160 bpm, 11.46% with BCFs absent, 0.63% with BCFs below 120 bpm and 1.29% with BCFs above 160 bpm.

III.6. DISCUSSION AND COMMENTS ON FREQUENCY RESULTS:

In our study we found that the frequency of oxytocin use in our setting was 3.28%.PIERRE BUEKENS, in his study on the over-medication of maternity care in developing countries, studied the frequency of three parameters: caesarean section, episiotomy and the use of oxytocin.With regard to the latter, it found high frequencies oxytocin use during the periods of effacement, dilation and expulsion in Africa, sometimes with rates of more than 20%, as in Saint Louis (Senegal) 32.9% and Bamako (Mali26%. We therefore say that obstetric interventions must be based on evidence, and interventions that are effective only for certain conditions. However, it is not clear that such a global epidemic exists, because studies have generally focused on one country or region [18].

AGE :

The mean age was 27.5 years, with extremes ranging from 14 to 4 years. In our study, we found that 28.66% or 45 parturients were aged between 20 and 24, followed by 25.47% or 43 parturients aged between 25 and 29. The same observation was also made by FOUDJET KOWA who found in his study that pregnant women in 18-34 age group had a frequency of 81.7% with an average age of 27.62. MAMADOU MOUSSA N'DIAYE found a frequency of 60.4% for almost the same age groups. This high representativeness was also found in the DHENYO ZABA study, and we agree with them that this age bracket corresponds to the period of full genital activity and not to the age bracket when there is a greater risk of requiring an oxytocin infusion for childbirth [7, 13, 5].

CIVIL STATUS :

We found that 94.909% or 149 pregnant women were married. The same finding was made by DHENYO in his study and he found that 68.7% of his respondents were married; and MAMADOU MOUSSA NDIAYE also made the same finding. We say that married women are more affected by this obstetric condition because they represented the highest proportion in our study. In our study, we found that most parturients were housewives with 83 cases (52.86%), followed by students with 34 cases (21.65%). The same observation was made by DHENYO in his study with a frequency of 37.7% and MAMADOU also made the same observation with a frequency of 64.2%. We also agree with MAMADOU that none these functions seems to be a determining factor in the need for oxytocin infusion during childbirth [5, 13].

PARITY :

We have noticed that primiparous and multiparous cows have almost the same frequency, with 43.94% for primiparous cows and 43.06% for multiparous cows. Large multiparous cows finished with 7.00%. MYLENE COLMANT in her study on syntocinon-directed labour in 2010 found 59% primiparous and 41% multiparous women and SANS-Caroline found 49.5% primiparous and 50.5% multiparous women. This discrepancy may confirm the hypothesis that the flow rate or use of oxytocin does not seem to be influenced by maternal age, gestational age, BMI or weight gain pregnancy, nor is there any difference between the duration of labour in primiparous and multiparous women in the presence of oxytocin infusion, as found by MYLENE [17].

INDICATIONS :

In terms of indications, we noted that hypokinesias had a higher frequency than the other indications with 42.64%, followed by MIU with 29.29% and RPM with 12.10%. In the study carried out by JULIA BLANCHOT, she found that late term came in first place with 32.6%, followed by LMP with 22.5%, while for CHIESA MOUTANDOU MBOUMBA S. LMP came in first place with 47%, followed by hypertension during pregnancy with 31.9% and UTI with 9.7%; KANGUDIA M. AND COL found that LMP came in first place with 32.6%, followed by UTI with 22.5%. Dysgravidia and post-maturity had 72% and the other indications only 28%. In spite of these differences in results, we think that this can be justified by the time and the different study environments, and in our study, we say that hypokinesias are due to uterine fibromyomas, diagnosed or not, given that this pathology is frequent in the black race and in women aged 35-50 years according to Labama L, and over 30 years according to Pierre et Marie Curie; For IMT, we believe that with the depravity of morals in our environment, the prevalence of transmission of infections (syphilis, etc.) is frequent and could be the cause of the disease.Finally, we also believe that advanced maternal age, multiparity and unfavourable socio-economic conditions may explain PMR [10, 4, 11,12 ,18].

COMPLICATIONS :

During our study we found that most of our respondents did not present complications either during or after the oxytocin infusion, i.e. 84.07% and 5.73% respectively. 3.82% failed oxytocin infusion; 3.18% hypertonia; 1.27% hyperkinesia and 1.91% fetal heart rhythm abnormalities. The majority of our respondents gave birth without complication; this can be explained firstly by the fact that the parturients arrived at the hospital with a favourable Bishop score and secondly by the effort made by the nursing staff in caring for the patients, even though the working conditions and technical facilities in our environments are deplorable. In her study, JULIA found that 25.3% of patients undergoing artificial labour induction for medical reasons underwent a caesarean section, with 5.6% for stagnation dilatation or failure, 64.4% for foetal anomaly (foetal heart rate anomalies), 1 case of cord procidence and 1 case of forehead presentation. PIERRE BWENKENS points out in his study that the administration of an excessive dose of oxytocin can cause hyperstimulation (which can even lead to spontaneous rupture of the membranes) and even uterine hypertonia. The same excessive dose of oxytocin is also incriminated in the genesis of foetal heart rate anomalies by JULIA, and we too join them in justifying these complications in our work, given that the same causes produce the same effects. The failures, as we have already pointed out, can be justified by the use of oxytocin infusion on a cervix that is in unfavourable conditions, i.e. a BISHOP score of less than 5. The risk is probably greater in developing countries such as ours, where the product is often administered without a pump controlling the speed of the intravenous infusion. MYLENE Supports the fact that the condition of the perineum depends on the rate of infusion, as a high rate of infusion is responsible for significant tearing of the perineum. Studies from West Africa and NEPAL suggest a higher risk fetal distress and neonatal morbidity associated with the use of oxytocin during labour [18, 17, 10].

DILATION AND ERASURE :

Dilatation and effacement are the few elements that can allow us to achieve the BISHOP score, even though these two parameters cannot allow us to achieve this score; but we can have an idea of what the score might be in certain parturients. In our study, 14.3% of parturients had dilatation of between 1-2 cm and 15.28% with effacement of between 0-30%. According to Berland M., although the duration of cervical dilation during labour depends on many factors: gestational age, parity, posture of the parturient, state of the membranes, height and orientation of the presentation this are essentially the The physical characteristics of the cervix, especially in the first phase of labour (2 to. In view of our results, we can say that some pregnant women may have had an unfavourable bishop score, which could explain the failures we recorded in our study, as supported by several authors (FOUDJET, HAS, LABAMA L..) [7, 8,12,].

CONCLUSION AND RECOMMENDATIONS

At the end of our retrospective study on childbirth by oxytocin infusion in Kisangani from January 2011 to December 31, 2012, the objectives of which were to determine the profile of pregnant women who had benefited from oxytocin infusion during labour and to identify accidents caused by this method of induction or maintenance of labour, Despite the limitations of our study and the difficulties encountered, our work has shown that our results are consistent with studies carried out by other researchers. Our study shows that 3.28% of deliveries in Kisangani are carried out by oxytocin infusion.

We can therefore assume that :

- The average age of the pregnant women who benefited from oxytocin infusion was 27.5 years, with extremes of age ranging from 14 to 41 years, and parturients aged 20-24 years were more numerous than others, with a frequency of 28.66%.
- The majority of our respondents lived in the commune of KABONDO (34.39%), were married (94.90%), housewives (52.86%), primiparous and multiparous respectively with 43.94% and 43.06% and had weak uterine contractions (45.94%).
- In our setting, hypokinesia is the most common indication for oxytocin infusion (42.64%), with more than half of our respondents achieving dilatation greater than or equal to 5cm (60.50%) and effacement greater than 80% (36.32%).
- These deliveries were uncomplicated in 84.07% of cases, with 5.73% involving perineal tears, 3.82% failures and 3.18% hypertonia.
- Hypokinesias were more frequent than the other indications with 42.64%, followed by MIU with 29.29% and RPM with 12.10%.

- primiparous and multiparous women have almost the same frequency, with 43.94% for primiparous women and 43.06% for multiparous women.
- 94.909% or 149 pregnant women were married.

RECOMMENDATIONS

➢ TO THE POLITICAL AND ADMINISTRATIVE AUTHORITIES

Equipping hospitals with essential equipment for better patient care, for example in our case: monitoring, volumetric pump for infusion of oxytocin.

➢ TO CARE STAFF

Always weigh up the advantages and disadvantages of infusing oxytocin before applying it; Always monitor this infusion (flow rate) once it has been placed and also monitor all the elements of the partogram to prevent any complications of origin.

➢ TO RESEARCHERS

We do not claim have said or done everything, which is why we are asking other researchers to continue their research in this area, where we have not covered every aspect.

BIBLIOGRAPHY

1. ANONYMOUS,THE CARE LINKED A CHILDBIRTH NORMAL:Guide guide. Report of group of borking group.64P

2. BERLAND, M., physiologie du déclenchement spontané du travail in collection tsunami, 2006, 205-21 1p.

3. BERNARD ET GENEVIEVE P., Dictionnaire médical pour les régions tropicales, Saint Paul, Kinshasa, 2002.

4. CHIESA MOUTANDOU-MBOUMBA S.,MOUNANGA M.,MAYI DECLENCHEMENT ARTIFICIEL DU TRAVAIL PAR LE INTRAVAGINAL MISOPROSTOL. Etude prospective au GABON chez 97 patientes de janvier 1997 à juin 1998, Médecine d'Afrique Noire : 1999, 46(12), PP 557.

5. DHENYO ZABA,B., Profil et prise en charge des gestantes porteuses de grossesse prolongée aux CUKIS, UNIKIS, D4 Kisangani, 2011 , unpublished

6. FATTORUSSO, V., RITTER, 0., oxytocin in: VADEMECUM CLINIQUE du diagnostic au traitement, 17th edition, I1I MASSON.

7. FOUDIET KOWA,R., L'utilisation du misoprostol dans la prise en charge des grossesses arrêtées dans le service de Gynécologie Obstétrique de l'hôpital GABRIEL TOURE à propos de 60 cas, université de BAMAKO, thèse de doctorat, BAMKO, 2005, 11 1p.(inédit).

8 HAUTE AUTORITE DE SANTE, Recommandation professionnelles Déclenchement artificiel du travail à partir de 37 semaines d'aménorrhée, France, 2008,2 1P.

9. JEAN-PATRICK, S. (eds), délivrance dirigée. Mécanique et Technique Obstétricales B., 3rd edition, 1994, pg607

10. JULIA BLANCHOT, artificial induction of labour at term at Port-Royal:

Evaluation of professional practices between 1999 and 2009 in the light of the HAS recommendations of 2008, Dissertation, Paris Descartes University, Paris, 2011,71P. (Unpublished).

11. KANGUDIA, M. et AL. Induction of labour in under-equipped environments, Congo Médical, no.15, 2004, pp 2325.

12. LABAMA LOKWA, B., Obstétrique du praticien, Presses de l'université de Kisangani, Kisangani, 2005.

13. MAMADOU MOUSSA NDIAYE, La mort fœtale in utéro à la maternité RENEE CISSE DHAMDALLAYE : Aspect clinique, épidémiologique et prise en charge, université de BAMAKO, thèse de doctorat, BAMAKO, 2003,95P. (Unédit).

14. MANGA, P., Obstetrics, University of Kindu, 1st doctorate course, Kindu, 2010, (unpublished).

15. MARINI djang'einga, R., Pharmacologie spéciale, université de Kisangani, cours de 1èdoctorat, Kisangani, 392P. (Unpublished).

16. MERGER, R., LEVY,). and MELCHIOR, J. Thérapeutiques médicamenteuses au cours du travail. In: précis d'obstétrique, 6th edition, Masson, 1995, pg478.

17. Mylène COLMANT, SYNTOCINON®-LED WORK:
Evaluation carried out at the Bar-le-DuUC maternity hospital, Université Henri-Poincare, Nancy I, dissertation, Nancy, 2010
,90OP.(unpublished).

18. PIERRE BUEKENS, La sur médication des soins aux mères dans les pays en développement, studies in HSOEP, University of North Carolina at Chapel Hill, USA, 2001, 13P. (Unpublished).

19. PIERRE et MARIE CURIE: Gynaecology, University of Paris VI, 2003, unpublished lecture.

20. SANS-CAROLINEAMNIOTOMY DURING LABOUR SPONTANE : Etude descriptive rétrospective à l'hôpital couple enfant du CHU de Grenoble, université JOSEPH FOURIER, dissertation, grenoble, 2012, 38p.Unpublished).

21. WEIN, P., Efficacy of different startingdoses of oxytocin for induction oflabor. ObstetGynecol, 1989; 74:863 - 868, in tsunami collection, 2006, pp 205-211.

WEBOGRAPHY

22. www.Bébépassion.com/accouchement/déctenchement12/11/ 2012 at 10pm

23. www.medical78.com/mat trigger.htm12/11/2012 at 10pm

24. www.gyneweb.fr/sources/Obstétrique/Concessus.htm15/11/ 2012at 10pm

25. www.pro.gyneweb.f15/11/2012

26. URL:http.www.guineegresse.info/index.php?id=14,10399,0,0, 1.0 14 /11/2012 at 8pm.

27. www.expobiologie.free.fr/ocytocne.htm 14/11/2012 at 10pm

28. http://blog.doctissimo.fr/info[...]e/articles/16/11/2012 at 8pm

29. http://www.unilim.fr/gynov/perinat/publc/infogrossesse/acc ouchement.htm12/12/201 at 5 pm

30. http://www.jsieurope.org/safem/cgi-bin/library.fcgi?e=p- 0safem--00-1-0-01040-11--1fr-5000---50-topic---01131-0011*07M!lIkffffffff00000000478f8d1e-0utfZz-8-0-0 a=d&jn=s2961f10/01/2013 at 7pm

TABLE OF CONTENTS

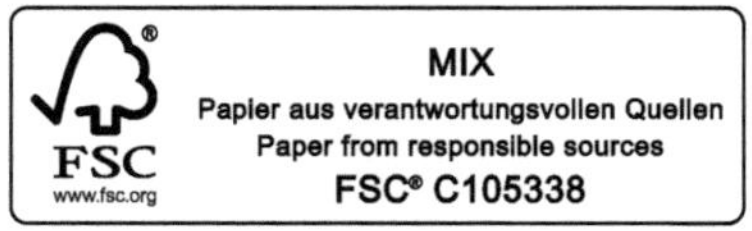

Printed by Books on Demand GmbH, Norderstedt / Germany